Moise Musa Wabula

Determinants of non-completion of the Children's Vaccination Schedule

Moise Musa Wabula

Determinants of non-completion of the Children's Vaccination Schedule

12 to 23 MONTHS in Kinshasa (Bandalungwa Health Zone)

ScienciaScripts

Imprint

Cover image: www.ingimage.com

This book is a translation from the original published under ISBN 978-620-3-41587-2.

Publisher:
Sciencia Scripts
is a trademark of
Dodo Books Indian Ocean Ltd. and OmniScriptum S.R.L publishing group

120 High Road, East Finchley, London, N2 9ED, United Kingdom
Str. Armeneasca 28/1, office 1, Chisinau MD-2012, Republic of Moldova, Europe
Managing Directors: Ieva Konstantinova, Victoria Ursu
info@omniscriptum.com

Printed at: see last page
ISBN: 978-620-8-55463-7

TABLE OF CONTENTS

DEDICATION

To you, my dear parents ***WABULA NGOZI BUKONGO Jean-Pierre and BITANGALO MUSA Régine****, the source of my life, for all the sacrifices you have made since my early childhood to help me become an independent person today. This work is a proof of your high sense of responsibility towards me, you initiated the path of school, which allowed me to be competitive among many others, please collect the fruit of your efforts.*

To you, my loving wife, ***NONDO ZABAKINGA Denise****, for so much love, support in the worst of times and patience during these two years of study when we gave up everything to go back to square one. Please find here all my attachment and my immeasurable consideration.*

To you, my dearest children, ***BITANGALO WABULA Plamédie*** *and* ***WABULA NGOZI, thank you*** *for the love you have always shown me, which has enabled me to be more than determined to accomplish this noble mission. Please find here a model to follow throughout your life, I leave you a legacy of perseverance, courage and determination.*

ACKNOWLEDGEMENTS

At the end of this master's degree course in Public Health, option: Intervention Epidemiology and Laboratory Management, we can pay homage to the creator of the universe, Almighty God, source of life, because everything is accomplished by his will.

None of this could have been achieved without the support of a number of eminent scientists, including the teaching and administrative staff of the Faculty of Medicine at the University of Kinshasa in general, and the staff of the Kinshasa School of Public Health in particular. We would like to express our sincere gratitude to them all.

Our deepest gratitude goes to the eminent ***Professor Dr MAPATANO MALA Ali****, who spared no effort in agreeing to supervise this dissertation. Despite his heavy workload, he accompanied us step by step like a father to ensure that this work met the requirements of the scientific world, with many comments and clarifications.work of this scale can be carried out without financial support and a partnership agreement, and so we pay a warm tribute to the American Government through its Disease Control and Prevention Agency "CDC Atlanta" and the Government of the Democratic Republic of Congo through its Directorate of Disease Control "DLM" for having made commitments by mutual agreement to ensure that the overall funding of our training at the School of Public Health at the University of Kinshasa is effective.*

We would also like to thank all the supervisors during these two years of training.

We must not forget to thank the health and political-administrative authorities of the ZS and the Bandalungwa commune, who agreed to allow this work to be carried out in their respective jurisdictions.

My thanks also go in particular to the family of ***Professor BULAIMU WITE NKATE MYANDA Augustin****, who accompanied me and my family here to Kinshasa.*

We would like to thank all our friends and acquaintances for having contributed in one way or another, both morally and materially, to achieve this work.Finally, we would like to thank all the colleagues in the FELTP family in general, and in the 3rd Cohort in particular, for the wonderful moments of joy, love and conviviality we have shared together. Let everyone, wherever they may be, know that we are infinitely grateful and that they are now part my extended family.

SUMMARY

INTRODUCTION

Vaccination has been shown to be the most effective way of fighting disease ever, and is one of the strategies for reducing morbidity and mortality, especially among children. In the DRC, there are still huge disparities in terms of vaccination coverage for children aged between 12 and 23 months, which hovers around 45%.The Bandalungwa HZ has also had low coverage over the last three years, at around 65%. This is why this study aimed identify the determinants of non-completion of the immunisation schedule in children aged 12 to 23 months in this health zone.

METHODOLOGY

We conducted an analytical cross-sectional study in the Bandalungwa HZ from 23 November to 23 December 2016, among 367 households with at least one child aged 12 to 23 months at the time of our survey. We estimated the proportion of fully vaccinated children (ECV) and children not fully vaccinated (ENCV). Bivariate analysis and logistic regression enabled us to identify the determinants of non-completion of the vaccination schedule. ORs with 95% CIs were used to measure the strength of association between the dependent variable and the independent variables.

RESULTS

Vaccination coverage was 41.4% (IC95%: 36-45). The determinants of non-completion of the vaccination schedule were: the availability of the vaccination card (ORA: 144.1; CI95% 33.74-615.74; p=0.00), the long waiting time at the vaccination site (0RA: 2.19; CI95%: 1.17-4.11; p< 0.05) and the high cost of the CPS session (ORA: 4.21; CI95%: 2.33-6.75; p=0.006).

CONCLUSION

The strategies for improving immunisation coverage in the Bandalungwa health zone could include keeping the immunisation card in good condition and making it available to the facilities that immunise, improving the organisation of immunisation sessions through training supervision and reducing the fees charged to mothers who bring their children to immunisation sessions.

***Key words**: completion, vaccination, schedule, Bandalungwa, Children aged 12 to 23 months.*

CHAPTER I

INTRODUCTION

1.1. Problem Statement

The World Health Organisation (WHO) points out that measles, poliomyelitis, diphtheria, hepatitis B, bacterial meningitis, rabies and tetanus, all vaccine-preventable diseases, cause a great deal of morbidity and disability that can be prevented by vaccination. **(1)**

It is currently estimated that 2 to 3 deaths a year neonatal tetanus and measles can be prevented by vaccination. By 2013, 129 countries had achieved DPT3 coverage of at least 90%. **(2)**

In 2014, around 86% (115 million) of infants worldwide received all three doses of the DTP vaccine. **(3)**

Despite progress in vaccination coverage worldwide over the last decade, disparities remain at national, regional and local level.

In 2014, WHO estimates show that 14% of infants worldwide were not covered by routine immunisation services, including the administration of DTP3. More than 60% of these children live in 10 , including South AfricaEthiopiaIndia, Indonesia, Iraq, Nigeria, Uganda, Pakistan, the Philippines and the Democratic Republic of Congo **(2)**.

The WHO recommends that priority be given to strengthening routine immunization worldwide, particularly in countries with the highest numbers of unimmunized children. Special efforts should be made to reach underserved populations, particularly in remote areas, poor urban settings, fragile states and conflict-affected regions **(3).**

In the Democratic Republic of Congo, the 2013-2014 DHS report reveals that 22% of children aged 12-23 months had been fully vaccinated according to information obtained from the vaccination record. **(4)** When the information provided by the mother is added, this percentage rises to 45%. Conversely, 6% of all children aged 12-23 months had not received any vaccinations at all. The remaining 49%, or one child in two, had therefore been partially vaccinated, while 41% had been fully vaccinated according to the recommended schedule, i.e. before the age of 12 months.A study carried out in Kinshasa on the knowledge, attitudes and practices of mothers of children aged 0-4 years also showed that vaccination coverage based on information recorded on the vaccination card was also low (37%), indicating a difference between the high level of knowledge and positive attitudes and the low coverage **(5).**The 2015 annual report of the Expanded Programme on Immunisation (EPI) notes that immunisation data low coverage for certain antigens, including measles, neonatal tetanus and polio **(6).**The results of routine EPI activities in the provincial city of Kinshasa in the first half of 2014 revealed that 12 health zones, namely: Bumbu, Kalami I, Lemba, Makala, Ngaba, Kingasani, MasinaI, Barumbu , Binza-Ozone, Kintambo , Lingwala and Bandalungwa, i.e. 34% of health zones had less than 80% vaccination coverage for the first dose of Pentavalent (DTP-Hep B-Hib). The data for the first half of 2014 show that the mothers of 20,916 children aged between 0 and 11 months, who were due to receive the first dose of DTP-HepB-Hib vaccine, did not attend the vaccination service. This situation resulted in a high proportion of unreached children (14.3%) in the 12 health zones. This represents an average of 116 unvaccinated children per health area, if we consider that each health area is made up of an average of 15 health areas **(7).**

The surveillance data for these 12 health zones in Kinshasa show an under-reporting of AFP cases compared with the last five years, with 20 cases reported out of 191 expected for 11 health zones, i.e. 31.4% of health zones in the first quarter of 2014; 20 zones having reported at least one case of measles, 5 cases of dengue fever, indigenous cases of yellow fever and cases imported from the epidemic that was raging in ANGOLA are reported on a daily basis and cases of paediatric bacterial meningitis (PBM) are reported here and there.**(7)**

The Bandalungwa HZ one of the HZs experiencing these problems. Vaccination coverage is low (65%) for all antigens combined (2015), and there is a risk of several if no action is taken, given the ever-increasing numbers of susceptible people.

1.2. LITERATURE REVIEW

1.2.1. General information on vaccination

a) Definition of vaccination

The word "vaccine" comes from the Latin vaccinus, meaning "relating to cows". But what do cows have to do with vaccines? The first vaccine was based on the wild smallpox virus, which infected both cows and humans **(8).**

Vaccination is a method of preventing certain microbial, viral or parasitic infections by inducing active immunity through the introduction into the body of preparations known as vaccines. **(9)**

A vaccine is a substance prepared from pathogenic microbes, viruses or parasites and toxins (killed, inactivated or attenuated) which, when inoculated, confers immunity to the individual against the corresponding germ. **(10)**

b) History of vaccination

200 years ago, Edward Jenner realised that cows contracted bovine smallpox, which is not very virulent, without ever contracting human smallpox. So he took the pathogen from the epidermal ooze of an infected cow, and injected the liquid into the arm of a healthy young boy. Six weeks later, Jenner injected him with the human smallpox virus. The young boy did not get the disease, and it was in this way that Dr Jenner discovered one of the fundamental principles of immunisation. **(8)**

But when we talk about vaccines, one image inevitably comes to mind: Louis Pasteur. In 1885, Pasteur was the first researcher to develop a vaccine against rabies. This was the first means of combating pathogens, and therefore certain infectious diseases, that could be used on a massive scale and administered systematically.

The principle behind vaccination was explained by Louis Pasteur and his colleagues Roux and Duclaux, following Robert Koch's work linking microbes and diseases. **(11)**

This discovery enabled him to improve the technique. His first vaccination was of a flock of sheep against cholera on 5 May 1881. The first human vaccination was that of a child against rabies on 6 June 1885 **(11)**.

Today, there is a great diversity and quantity vaccines. This multiplicity of vaccines is explained by advances in vaccine manufacturing techniques. Scientists are improving existing vaccines and creating new ones to increase the protection they offer our bodies and reduce the risks. **(12)**

Key dates in the development of the main vaccines

- **1796:** Edward Jenner discovered the smallpox vaccine. Thanks to this discovery, the smallpox virus was eradicated.

- **1879:** Louis Pasteur discovers the vaccine against hen cholera;
- **1885**: Louis Pasteur explains the principle of vaccination and discovers the rabies vaccine;
- **1888**: Frenchmen André Chantemesse and Fernand Widal discover the typhoid fever vaccine;
- **1913**: Emil Adolf von Behring unveils the diphtheria vaccine.
- **1921**: Albert Calmette and Camille Guérin develop a vaccine against tuberculosis called BCG.
- **1927**: The tetanus is created by Pierre Descombey and Gaston Ramon.
- **1935**: Leslie Gardner develops a pertussis vaccine.
- **1944**: Thomas Francis Jr. creates a vaccine against influenza.
- **1949**: John Franklin Engers, Fred Robbins and Thomas Weller discover the mumps vaccine.
- **1953**: Jonas Salk produces the polio vaccine
- **1960**: John Franklin Engers develops a measles vaccine **(12)**

c) Vaccination coverage

Vaccination coverage is the proportion of people vaccinated in a given population at a given time. Its measurement is necessary to assess the effectiveness of any vaccination programme and to determine the degree of protection of a population against an infectious disease. In a given population, vaccination coverage is the ratio between the number of people correctly vaccinated and the total number of people who should have been vaccinated. For a vaccine requiring several doses, the term "one dose" is used.
"These include "two doses, "three doses" and "booster". **(13)**

d) Vaccination schedule :

The minimum vaccination schedule recommended in the DRC and adopted by the WHO includes BCG at birth, 3 doses of OPV, 3 doses of pentavalent, 3 PCV13, at 6th , $10^{(th)}$) and 14th weeks, currently a dose of IPV at 14th week and measles vaccine and yellow fever vaccine are recommended at $9^{(th)}$) month **(14)**.

e) Immunity

Immunity is the body's ability to defend itself against an infectious attack (bacteria, virus or parasite) or a given disease. **(15)**

ANTIGEN: Substance which the immune system recognises as foreign and which induces the formation of specific antibodies.

ANTIBODY: Any substance present naturally or produced in the body under the action of an antigen and which has the property of reacting specifically against this antigen. Antibodies are proteins secreted by cells called plasma cells, derived from B lymphocytes. Plasma antibodies are closely linked to certain globulins (immunoglobulins). The terms antibodies and immunoglobulins are often used synonymously **(16).**

Active immunization :

Active immunisation is an immune response by the body's antibodies to inoculated pathogens (vaccines). This response does not appear for some time, but the protection is long-lasting.

Passive immunisation :

Passive immunisation is the administration of foreign immunoglobulins, already active against the pathogen, to a recipient. It occurs without any reaction of the body itself. It is rapid but short-lived. It is often used in association with active immunisation when a person is exposed to the pathogen **(16).**

1.2.2. Vaccination situation

Immunisation is recognised worldwide as one of the most effective measures for preventing mortality, morbidity and complications of infectious diseases in children. **(17)**

Vaccination coverage indicates the proportion of the target population that has received the required doses a vaccine against a preventable disease **(18).** It is an important indicator of population health and a good reflection of susceptibility to vaccine-preventable diseases1 (VPDs) **(17,19).** It can also be used to assess the accessibility of health services and vaccination-related interventions, and provide a rapid assessment of whether health services are improving or deteriorating. As high levels of immunisation coverage are required to achieve the goals of reducing vaccine-preventable diseases, it is essential to monitor the various measures of immunisation coverage on an ongoing basis.

The success of vaccination programmes should not be taken for granted, as their success depends on the confidence of the public and health professionals.

Vaccination in Africa dates back to the pre-independence era, when mobile teams were used to carry out mass vaccinations to combat epidemics such as smallpox and yellow fever **(20)**.

The recent survey of vaccination coverage in 2012 in the DRC shows inequalities in vaccination coverage between the different antigens, provinces and within the same province between health zones. Coverage varies from 73.2% to 97.3% for BCG, from 54% to 87.7% for VAR, and from 50.2% to 93.9% for DTP3 at national level. For children who have received all vaccines, coverage varies between 37.9% and 85.2%. **(6)**

The same survey found that lack of information, lack of motivation and the distance between the vaccination site and the child's home were the main reasons why children were not vaccinated. **(6)**

1.2.3. Determinants of vaccination

Several factors have been described in the literature to explain the non-completion and completion of the childhood immunisation schedule (21, 23, 25, 27). Socio-demographic characteristics, the organisation of the healthcare system and the knowledge, attitudes and practices of mothers are among the groups of factors most frequently cited.

Socio-demographic characteristics

- **Characteristics specific to children**

A study carried out in the Dschang district of Cameroon in 2013 showed that the first siblings to be born completed their immunisation schedule compared with subsequent births. **(21)**

Similarly for the child's place of birth, being born in a medical facility plays a major role in immunisation status compared with children born at home, respectively 87.9% and 7.7% (**21**).

This difference can be explained by the low level of awareness and negligence on the part of parents (forgetfulness of appointments 33.2%, and lack of time 40.3%) **(22)**. To remedy this Ndeye et al. recommended raising awareness and requiring school-age children to carry vaccination records with them. **(23)**

- **Level of education of mothers responsible for children aged 12 to 23 months**

Low levels of education play a major role in children not completing their immunisation schedule (21, 24, 26). However, a study conducted in Nigeria proves the opposite. It found that children born to illiterate parents had completed their immunisation schedule. vaccination schedule. **(27)** This contradiction would be justified by the availability of these mothers due to lack of work, as most literate mothers are often busy and avoid appointments to complete their children's vaccination schedule. In addition, other studies in West Africa have shown that parental education plays no role in the completion of the immunisation schedule. **(28)**

Parental occupation, religious beliefs and socio-economic level

A study carried out in Algeria on the vaccination status of children during the P.A.S period in 2015 showed a significant association between the non-completion of the child's vaccination schedule and the parents' occupation, religious beliefs and customs. On the other hand, it showed that children of unemployed parents had not completed their children's vaccination schedule. **(28)**

In addition, it has been noted that low parental income is a barrier to some households completing the vaccination schedule **(29).**

In the same study (24), the results showed that the factors that have a positive and independent influence on vaccination are the child's first rank in the sibling group, having a regular source of vaccination, receiving all vaccines free of charge and a high family income.

Non-compliance with the vaccination schedule

In the study conducted in Côte d'Ivoire in 2008 **(30),** 14% of mothers suggested that non-compliance with the schedule was one of the causes of non-vaccination. However, in some cases, 31% of mothers had not been informed of the need to return for further doses, and 32% cited ignorance of the need to have their children vaccinated.

Health service factors

Travel the distance from home to the vaccination site and back:

A study carried out in Mozambique (**31**) in 2003 showed that the distance children had to travel was the main reason why they were not vaccinated. In Chad in 2012, 19% of mothers mentioned this (**32**).

The study carried out in Senegal in 2005 found that 71% of children were fully vaccinated.

Vaccine unavailability :

Low vaccination coverage among children was also described as a contributing factor. In many countries, vaccination sites were often out of stock of the vaccine. This was the case in Côte d'Ivoire, where 75% of mothers cited this as a reason for not vaccinating **(30),** 10% in Chad in 2012 **(32)** and 13% of mothers in Benin **(27).**

Waiting times and reception at the vaccination site

In their studies on the non-completion of children's immunisation schedules, some authors have found a statistically significant link between long waiting times at the vaccination and poor reception at the vaccination site. This was the case in Bushidi in the DRC in 2012. **(33).** Baonga S et al in Cameroon in 2012. **(34)**

Mothers' knowledge, skills and practices regarding vaccination

Low vaccination coverage has led some authors to study the population's behaviour towards vaccination. In some countries, the drop in vaccination coverage has been attributed to a lack of knowledge of the vaccination schedule on the part of some mothers (35) and a lack of awareness of vaccine-preventable diseases (36). Mothers' low level of knowledge about vaccination has been cited by several authors as one of the main factors predicting non-completion of the child's vaccination schedule. (33, 34, 37,38)

The study carried out by Mapatano et al (**5**) and that Batumbo **(39)** showed that mothers had positive attitudes to vaccination, but had a low level of knowledge of the vaccination schedule in force in the DRC. Furthermore, RIMPLE et al (40) and Matango (41) showed that refusal of vaccination was greater among certain mothers belonging to certain religions or because of idolatry.In addition, good practice has been observed for mothers who have already experienced the severity of MEV (5,40)

Fear of side effects:

It has been noted that the perceived risk side-effects following vaccination is a handicap for mothers taking part in the vaccination programme. (5,35).

In 2012 the survey carried out in the Democratic Republic of Congo revealed the reasons for non-vaccination in descending order: (42)

1.3. QUESTION BY RECHERE

In the majority of Kinshasa's health zones, an improvement in vaccination coverage has been noted over the last 5 years, whereas it is still unclear in **the Bandalungwa** health zone, vaccination coverage remains low, not exceeding 65% over the last 3 years. This is why we want to know what factors might explain this low vaccination coverage,In Figure 1, the conceptual model shows us the relationships that demonstrate a link between the independent variables and the dependent variable as explained in the problem statement and the literature review.

Poorly trained staff
Presence of MAPI
Poor reception at the vaccination service
Long waiting times at the vaccination service
Remote vaccination site
High cost of vaccination service
Low household income
Mother's low level of education
Religious beliefs
Lack of confidence in vaccination
Busy mother
Young age of mother
Single mother
Poor maintenance of the cold chain
Poor vaccine administration
Not familiar with the vaccination
Poor geographical accessibility
Poor economic access to vaccination services
Low level of knowledge among mothers about vaccination
Mothers' poor attitude to vaccination
Mothers' poor vaccination practices
Poor organisation of vaccination service
No Completion of vaccination schedule Children aged 12 to 23 months

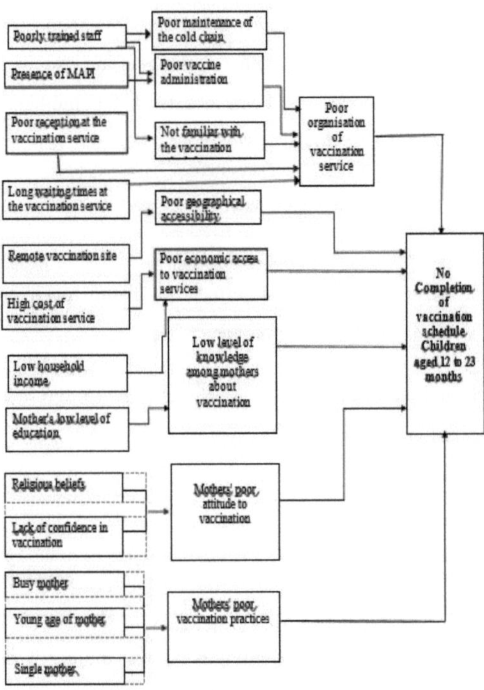

Figure 1: Conceptual model

1.4. HYPOTHESES

1. The poor quality service organisation assessed by mothers responsible children aged 12 to 23 months is associated with non-completion of the vaccination schedule

2. Low level of knowledge is associated with failure to complete the vaccination schedule,

3. Poor attitude to vaccination among mothers responsible for children aged 12 to 23 months is associated with non-completion of the vaccination schedule

4. Poor practices by mothers of children aged 12 to 23 months are associated with non-completion of the vaccination schedule

GOAL

Contribute to improving the demand for services and vaccination coverage in the BANDALUNGWA health zone.

1.5. OBJECTIVES

1.5.1. GENERAL OBJECTIVE

To determine the factors associated with non-completion of the routine immunisation schedule in children aged 12 to 23 months in the Bandalungwa HZ from 2014 to 2015.

1.5.2. SPECIFIC OBJECTIVES :

1. Describe the socio-demographic and economic characteristics of households with children aged 12 to 23 months in the Bandalungwa health zone;

2. Determine the vaccination coverage of children aged 12 to 23 months who lived in the Bandalungwa health zone during 2014-2015.

3. To determine the quality of the organisation of services for parents responsible children aged 12 to 23 months;

4. Identify the determinants of non-completion of the immunisation schedule for children aged 12 to 23 months in the Bandalungwa health zone.

5. To determine the knowledge, attitudes and practices of parents of children aged 12 to 23 months in the Bandalungwa Health Zone.

CHAPTER II

METHODOLOGY

2.1. Study framework

We conducted our study in the Bandalungwa health zone, located in the Lukunga health district, in the commune of the same name.

The health zone is limited:

- To the north via the Kokolo ZS ;
- To the south via the Selembao ZS ;
- To the east via the Ngiri Ngiri SCA
- To west, via Binza Ozone and Kintambo HZs

It covers an area of 6.82 km^2, with a population density of **21,581** inhabitants/km^2.
It has an estimated population of **203089** inhabitants (2015 census) spread over 8 health areas, with a population aged between 12 and 23 months of **6093** (3%)

2.2. Type study

We carried out a cross-sectional study study by administering a pre-texted questionnaire mothers children aged between 12 and 23 months.

2.3. Study period

The study began on 23 November 2016 and ended on 23 December 2016.

2.4. Target population and sampling

The study population consisted of all children aged between 12 and 23 months at the time of the survey and who had been resident in the Bandalungwa health zone for one year for children aged 12 months and two years for children aged 23 months.

2.5. Inclusion

Our study included

• Households with children born between 15 October 2014 and 15 September 2015, i.e. those aged between 12 and 23 months on the date of our survey and who lived in the ZS during that period.

2.6. Exclusion criteria

• Mothers of children aged 12 to 23 months who did not give their consent and those who did not have children eligible for our study.

2.7. Sample size

We used the standard WHO cluster sampling protocol to assess EPI vaccination coverage.

$$n \geq Z2 \ . p.q.d2$$

• nsample size

• z: parameter related to the alpha risk of error. We used the value Z= 1.96 for a risk of error fixed at 5%.

• p: proportion of children not vaccinated or not fully vaccinated in Kinshasa 32% (according to the RDC EDS 2013-2014 report)

• q: complement of p (100-32= 68%)

• d: desired precision

q = 1-0,32 = 0,68 ;z= 1.96

$n \geq$ **1, 96^2x 0,32x0,68 =3340,05^2**

To compensate for the non-responses, we added 10% to our sample size, i.e. 34 mothers responsible for children aged 12 to 23 months, which led us to 368. After rounding 370 mothers.

2.8. Sampling technique

Table II: Distribution children to be surveyed by health area in the Bandalungwa health zone

AS	Pop 2015	Proportion	No. of children to be surveyed/AS
ADOULA	33013	0,16	60
BISENGO	28426	0,14	52
KASA VUBU	6803	0,30	12
LINGWALA	20713	0,10	38
LUBUDI NORTH	20635	0,10	35
LUBUDI SUD	20635	0,10	36
LUMUMBA	39591	0,19	70
MAKELELE	33273	0,16	60
Total ZS	203089		367
Sample size	367		

We used cluster sampling to investigate the determinants of non-completion of the immunisation schedule for children 12 to 23 months among 370 mothers/caretakers in the Bandalungwa health zone.The SZ is made up 8 health areas comprising 46 streets/ avenues which were considered as clusters. Sampling was at three levels; In the first stage, 37 streets/aisles were selected at random from the total number of streets in the ZS, and within each street/aisle, after listing all the households, 10 households were selected random, giving us 370 households surveyed, each with an eligible child.

In the second degree, in the streets/avenues :

• The starting point was determined by a random choice direction.

• And then we went from one household to the next in the chosen direction until we had 10 eligible children.

In the third stage, if there was more than one child aged between 12 and 23 months in each household, a single child was drawn at random from among the eligible children.

2.9. Data collection tools and techniques

We used a semi-structured questionnaire developed, tested and validated by the WHO in the Democratic Republic of Congo (DRC) during the immunisation coverage survey organised in 2015. We interviewed 370 mothers of children aged between 12 and 23 months, to obtain information on their children's vaccination status and the reasons why they had not been vaccinated. We also looked for BCG scars on the left arm of each child.

2.10 .Complete list of variables

Dependent variable

The dependent variable is non-completion of the vaccination schedule

Independent variables

The independent variables selected are :

- Socio-demographic and economic characteristics of mothers ;
- Mothers' knowledge, attitudes and practices regarding vaccination ;
- The organisation of vaccination services; and
- Geographical accessibility of mothers responsible for children aged 12 to 23 months in the Bandalungwa HZ in 2016.

Operational definition of variables

1. Socio-demographic and economic factors of mothers responsible for children aged 12 to 23 months

- **Age**: age respondents at last birthday, by calculating age at birth up to survey date, quantitative variable (In years≤ 24 years: young age, ≥25 years: adult age)
- **Sex**: nominal qualitative variable (1. male, 2. female)

- **Mother's marital status**: nominal qualitative variable which determines the marital status of the mother responsible for a child aged 12 to 23 months (single, monogamous married, polygamous married, common-law, widowed, divorced).
- **Mother's level of education**: ordinal qualitative variable, expressing the highest level of

education attained by the mother responsible for the child aged 12 to 23 months (no level, primary, secondary and tertiary/university).

- **Mother's occupation**: nominal qualitative variable, which defines the occupation of the mother of the child aged 12 to 23 months at the time of our survey (housewife, shopkeeper, civil servant, private civil servant, no occupation, others to be specified).
- **Religion**: qualitative variable indicating the church attended by the mother responsible for the child aged 12 to 23 months (no religion, Catholic, Protestant, Kimbanguist, Muslim, revivalist church, Jehovah's Witnesses, other).
- **Index of socio-economic level**: (API index = adjusted poverty index) a composite variable that determines the socio-economic level of households based on whether or not they own certain household goods (tap water, internal toilet, permanent electricity, vehicle, flat-screen TV, refrigerator, tiled house). The index was calculated by summing the goods owned. The most affluent households (possession of these 7 goods, high level) and the least affluent households (low level) were those that had less than these 7 household goods.
- **Socio-economic level of people in households**: quantitative variables measured using the indicator (expenditure per person per day). Information daily household expenditure was collected in Congolese francs. The variables were grouped into two categories: people living below the poverty line (if expenditure is less than 6,000 Congolese francs, equivalent to 5 US dollars) and people living above the poverty line (if the expenditure is less than 6000 Congolese francs equivalent to 5 US dollars)

2. Socio-demographic characteristics of children aged 12 to 23 months

- **Gender of the child**: qualitative variable reflecting the physical and constitutive differences between children. It had two modalities: male and female.
- **Age**continuous quantitative variable ranging from 12 to 23 months.

3. Factors linked to organisation of health services (respondents' point of view)

- **Waiting time at the vaccination service**: quantitative ordinal variable which measures the time (per hour) between the arrival of the mother of the child at the vaccination site and the start of the vaccination. It was grouped into two categories (≤ 1 hour, normal waiting time) and (> 1 hour, long waiting time).
- **Reception at the vaccination site**: dichotomous variable expressing the level of courtesy shown by the health staff to the mother of the child. There were two modes: good and bad reception.
- **Vaccine availability at the vaccination site**: nominal qualitative variable expressing the

availability or non-availability of vaccination either due to vaccine stock shortage lack of cold chain (CDF): It had two modes (absence of at least one antigen, presence of all antigens.

- **ABIP history**: qualitative variable providing information on the occurrence of certain signs after the child had been vaccinated. It had two modes, yes, if at least one sign present, no if no sign was present.

4. Geographical and financial accessibility

- **Distance from home to vaccination site**: quantitative variable reflecting the walking time (per hour) between the household and the vaccination site. It was grouped into two categories: more than an hour (long distance) and less than an hour (normal distance).

- **Cost of CPS sessions**: qualitative variable assessing the cost of access to the CPS session, with two modalities high cost (more than one US dollar, normal: less than one US dollar)

5. Knowledge, attitudes and practices

- **Level of knowledge**: composite variable which assesses the degree to which the mother surveyed is informed about VPDs, the vaccination schedule, the benefits of vaccination, and the consequences of not vaccinating her children. We considered an acceptable level of knowledge, if she was able to name 5 VEMs, an advantage of vaccination and the consequences of not vaccinating her children. of vaccination, a consequence of vaccination and 5 appointments in the vaccination calendar and the low level, if it did not meet one of the 4 criteria.

- **Attitude**: composite variable assessing the child's mother' apprehension about vaccination. In this study, the mother of a child aged 12 to 23 months was considered to have a favourable attitude if she considered the vaccine to be protective, agreed to have her child vaccinated at a distance of more than one hour's walk and agreed to have her child vaccinated to protect him or her against EVD. The mother of a child aged 12 to 23 months was considered to have a favourable attitude if she met all 3 criteria, and an unfavourable attitude if she did not meet any of the 3 criteria.

- **Practices**: composite variables which assess the actions taken by the mother with regard to her child's vaccination. In our study, the mother of a child aged 12 to 23 months was considered to have good practices if her child was fully vaccinated and presented the vaccination card when the interviewers visited. And bad practice if the mother of the child aged 12 to 23 months did not meet one of the two criteria.

Operational definitions

• Valid coverage: this is when the vaccination has met the minimum date (validity criterion) in terms of the required age (according to the calendar) and the intervals between doses;

• Vaccination according to the card: this is when the mother presents an official EPI document recording the date of vaccination;

• Vaccination status: vaccination status a target child in relation to vaccine doses

• Drop-out: Any target child who, at some point, has used vaccination services and who, for various reasons, has not continued.

• Lost to follow-up: situation of a child who has had at least one contact with the vaccination services but who has not completed his or her vaccination series within the required timeframe before his or her first birthday.

• Missed vaccination opportunities: this is when a child passes through a health facility and does not receive all the doses of vaccine he/she was supposed to receive at that time;

• Corrected missed opportunities: this is when a child has finally received the vaccination concerned at a subsequent visit;

• Uncorrected missed opportunities: this is when the child has not received the missed doses in subsequent sessions;

• Fully vaccinated child (ECV): if the child has received 1 dose of BCG at birth, 3 doses of DTP-HepB-Hib/VPO/PCV-13 from 6 weeks of age and who respects the 4-week interval between doses and 1 dose of VAR/VAA at 9 months of age.

• Child not fully vaccinated (ENCV): this is a child who has either been insufficiently vaccinated, has not been vaccinated or has not been reached by the vaccination service within the required time and in the required doses. **(9)**

Study parameter Vaccination coverage

We estimated vaccination coverage by antigen. Table II: Determination variables or parameters of interest in the Bandalungwa Health Zone 2015.

Table III: Determination of variables of interest in the Bandalungwa Health Zone 2015.

Parameter	Determination
Valid coverage(%)	Number of children fully vaccinated (map/total number of children surveyed)
Gross coverage (%)	Number children who received all doses of vaccine (card) regardless of the schedule / Total number children surveyed.
Coverage coverage (%)	Number of eligible children who have received BCG (presence of record book, vaccination scar or card) / Total number of children surveyed.
Coverage coverage DTP 1 (%)	Number eligible children who received DTC 1 (booklet) / Total number of children surveyed.
Coverage DTP3 vaccination coverage (%)	Number of children aged 12 to 23 months who received the DTP3 (booklet) / Total number of children surveyed.
Coverage coverage (%)	Number of eligible children who received the VAR (booklet/total number of children surveyed)
Drop-out rate	(Number of children who received DTP1 - Number of children who received DTP3) / Number of children who received DTP1

4.11. Collection itself

Before collecting the data, we first obtained the approval of the local authorities (the mayor of the Bandalungwa commune and the Bandalungwa Chief Medical Officer). Data collection was carried out by a team of six interviewers and a supervisor, since on average it took a maximum of one hour to complete a questionnaire, and each interviewer completed five questionnaires per day. This brought us ten days of data collection.As far as the profile of the interviewers concerned, we decided on at least a state diploma or higher. And for the supervisor, we took into account a graduate or licentiate level experience in community surveys. The interviewers were trained at BCZS over three days, two of which were devoted to the andragogical exchange of the tool through simulation tests, and one day to pre-testing the tool in the field.

4.12. Data processing and analysis

After data collection, the questions were grouped avenue/cluster and by health area (HA). But before the actual processing, we carried out a quality control of the data to check for consistency and compliance with numbering and coding.The data were entered using Epi data software and exported to SPSS. for analysis. Proportions calculated for the categorical variables with their 95% confidence intervals. Bivariate analysis was performed to determine the associations between categorical variables and non-completion of the childhood immunisation schedule.Logistic regression was used to obtain adjusted Odds ratios with their 95% confidence intervals and significance intervals for each variable in order to measure the strength of association and to identify the factors associated with non-completion of the childhood immunisation schedule.

4.13. Ethical considerations

We have requested written authorisation from the ethics committee. The participants fully briefed on the aims, objectives and importance of this study improving vaccination coverage in the Bandalungwa health zone.Given the age of the child, we have provided their carers with as much information as possible about how the child was selected to take part in the study. We explained that participation in the study was voluntary, and that they could terminate the study at any time without any prejudice. We had informed the children's guardians that the identity of their children would be kept confidential to the extent permitted by law. Finally, we have them with a telephone number and a physical address so that they can contact us if they have any problems.

CHAPTER III

PRESENTATION OF RESULTS

This chapter presents the main results obtained from the survey of mothers responsible for children aged 12 to 23 months in the Bandalungwa HZ. These results, organised in the form of tables and figures, cover the following points:

1. the socio-demographic and economic characteristics of the mothers surveyed
2. Vaccination coverage ;
3. The proportion of incompletely vaccinated children ;
4. The knowledge, attitudes and practices of the mothers surveyed
5. Factors influencing non-completion of the vaccination schedule.

3.1. Socio-demographic characteristics of mothers of children aged 12 to 23 months

Table V. **Socio-demographic characteristics of mothers of children aged 12 to 23 months in the Bandalungwa HZ.**

Mothers of fully vaccinated children				
Variables				
	No		Yes	
Categories	Workforce	(%)	Workforce	(%)
Age of respondents	n =204		n=148	
<18	7	3,4	0	0,0
18 à 25	45	22,2	26	17,6
26 à35	104	50,9	88	59,4
>35	48	23,5	34	23,0
Marital status	n =211		n=152	
Single	52	24,6	27	17,8
Married monogamy	148	70,2	117	77,0
Married polygamy	4	1,9	4	2,6
Divorced, widowed, separate	6	2,8	3	2,0
Other	1	0,5	1	0,6
Religion	n= 211		n=152	
No	6	2,8	0	0,0
Catholic	43	20,4	45	29,6
Protestant	18	8,5	26	17,1
Kimbanguist	11	5,2	11	7,2
Muslim woman	6	2,8	0	0,0
Church of revival	112	53,2	64	42,2
Jehovah's Witness	6	2,8	2	1,3
Other	9	4,3	4	2,6
Level of study	n=211		n=152	
No	2	0,9	0	0,0
primary	63	29,8	16	10,5
Secondary	122	57,9	112	73,7
Superior or University	24	11,4	24	15,8
Profession	n=211		n=152	
Housekeeper	95	45,1	81	53,3
Retailer	30	14,2	26	17,1
Civil servant	14	6,6	8	5,3
Civil servant	22	10,4	17	11,2
No profession	50	23,7	19	12,5
Other	0	0,0	1	0,6

Table V shows that the 25-35 and >35 age groups accounted for 50.9% and 23.5% respectively of mothers who had not completed their children's immunisation schedule. On the other hand, 59.4% of mothers aged 26 to 35 and 23% of mothers aged >35 completed their children's vaccination schedule.

In terms of marital status, mothers married in monogamy were in the lead, followed by single mothers, with 70.2% and 24.6% respectively for those who had not completed their children's vaccination schedule, and 77% for those married in monogamy and 17.8% for single mothers.

Table v shows that 112 mothers from the revivalist churches (53.2%) and 43 mothers from the Catholic church (20.4%) had not completed their children's vaccination schedule. On the other hand, 64 mothers from the revivalist church (17.63%) and 45 mothers from the Catholic church (12.4%) had fully vaccinated their children.

In terms of level of education, secondary education is in the lead, followed by primary education, with 57.9% and 29.8% respectively for mothers who have not completed their children's vaccination schedule and those who have completed their children's vaccination schedule. The figures are 73.7% for secondary education and 15.8% for higher education or university.

Housewives and women without a profession, who account for 45.1% and 23.7% respectively, are in the lead for those who have not completed their children's vaccination schedule, and for those who have completed their children's vaccination schedule. Housewives are followed by shopkeepers, with 53.3% and 17.1% respectively.

Socio-economic characteristics of mothers of children aged 12 to 23 months

Table VI: Distribution mothers according to ownership of certain household goods.

	Fully vaccinated children			
Household goods	No		Yes	
	n= 210	%	n= 152	%
Tap water				
Yes	177	84,3	129	84,9
No	38	18,1	23	15,1
Internal Toilet				
Yes	43	20,5	74	48,7
No	172	81,9	78	51,3
Permanent Electricity				
Yes	146	69,5	121	79,6
No	69	32,9	31	20,4
Vehicle				
Yes	35	16,7	24	15,8
No	180	85,7	128	84,2
Flat TV				
Yes	144	68,6	121	79,6
No	71	33,8	31	20,4
Fridge				
Yes	137	65,2	97	63,8
No	78	37,1	55	36,2
Tiled house				
Yes	69	32,9	79	52,0
No	146	69,5	73	48,0

Table VI shows that the proportion of mothers of children aged 12 to 23 months who were not in possession of certain household goods was higher in the ENCVs than in the ECVs. It shows that failure to complete the immunisation schedule for children aged 12 to 23 months was associated with non-possession of certain household goods, i.e. d. children from deprived families are more likely not to complete their children's immunisation schedule.

3.2. Vaccination coverage

Table VII: Vaccination coverage by antigen of children aged 12 to 23 months according to vaccination card, Bandalungwa HZ, 2016.

Antigens	Workforcen= 367	Percentage
BCG	195	53,1
PENTA1	204	55,6
PENTA3	176	48,0
VPO3	178	48,5
PVC-13	163	44,4
VAR	162	44,1
VAA	160	43,6

Table VII shows that vaccination coverage for all antigens was lower than that of the HZ and the national standard. The BCG-VAR and Penta1-3 drop-out rates were 16.9% and 13.7% respectively.

Table VIII. Vaccination coverage by antigen of children aged 12 to 23 months the Bandalungwa Health Zone according to map and mothers' declarations.

Antigens	Number n= 367	Percentage
BCG	291	79,3
PENTA1	232	61,3
PENTA3	199	50,7
VPO3	225	54,2
PVC-13	186	46,6
VAR	243	66,2
VAA	242	65,9

Table VIII shows that vaccination coverage for all antigens is still lower than in the health zone and the national norm. The BCG-VAR and Penta 1-3 drop-out rates remain high compared with the norm, at 16.48% and 11.34% respectively.

3.3. Proportion of children Fully Vaccinated in Bandalungwa Health Zone

Vaccination coverage for children aged 12 to 23 months is shown in the table below

Table IX: Proportion of children fully vaccinated according to map and mothers' declarations.

Features	n=367	%
Mothers of children aged 12 to 23 months with card available	212	57,8
ECV on the basis of the card	150	40,9
ECV on the basis of the card+ History of vaccination	152	41,4

Of the 367 mothers responsible for children aged 12 to 23 months questioned, 212 (57.8 ± 7%, IC95% 50.8-64.8) had their children's vaccination available. The proportion of ECVs was 40.9 ± 7% (IC95% 33.9-47.9) on the basis of the vaccination card, and 41.4 ± 7% (IC95% 34.4-48.4) on the basis of both methods.

Table X: Breakdown of immunisation coverage of children aged 12 to 23 months by Health Area in Bandalungwa HZ, 2016.

HEALTH AREAS		INCOMPETENT VACCINES		FULLY VACCINATED	
	n	Workforce	%	Workforce	%
ADOULA	60	32	53	28	47
BISENGO	52	19	37	33	63
KASA VUBU	12	10	83	2	17
LINGWALA	39	14	36	25	64
LUBUDI NORTH	37	17	46	20	54
LUBUDI SUD	38	23	61	15	39
LUMUMBA	69	52	75	17	25
MAKELELE	60	48	80	12	20
Total	367	215	59	152	41

The health districts of Kasavubu and Makelele come top with 83% and 80% respectively of children who have not completed their immunisation schedule, while the health districts of Lingwala and Bisengo have 64% and 63% respectively of children who have completed their immunisation schedule.

Table XI. Vaccination coverage by antigen and AS Bandalungwa Health Zone, 2016

Health areas Population surveyed Antigens

BCG Penta1 Penta3 VAR

	n	Workforce	%	Workforce	%	Workforce	%	Workforce	%
ADOULA	60	50	83,3	48	80,0	35	58,3	43	71,7
BISENGO	52	45	86,5	42	80	38	73,1	40	76,9
KASA VUBU	12	10	83,3	4	33,3	2	16,7	7	58,3
LINGWALA	38	34	87,2	32	82,1	29	74,4	30	76,9
LUBUDI NORTH	35	31	86,1	31	86,1	21	58,3	28	77,8
LUBUDI SUD	36	28	73,7	22	57,9	19	50,0	21	55,3
LUMUMBA	71	50	72,5	26	37,7	24	34,8	40	58,0
MAKELELE	60	42	70,0	19	31,7	17	28,3	33	55,0

Table XI shows that the AS of Lingwala had 87.2% coverage for BCG, followed by the AS of Bisengo (86.5%), for Penta1 , the AS of Lubudi Nord was in the lead (86.1%) followed by that of Lingwala (82,1%), for Penta3, the AS of Lingwala was still in the lead (74.4%) followed by that of Bisengo (73.1%) and finally for the VAR, the AS of Lubudi Nord was in first place (77.8%) followed by that of Lingwala (76.9%).

3.4. Knowledge, attitudes and practices of mothers of children aged 12 to 23 months Bandalungwa Health Zone

Table XII. Knowledge of mothers responsible for children aged 12 to 23 monthsvaccine-preventable diseases

	Fully vaccinated children			
MEV	No		Yes	
	n= 215	%	n= 149	%
Polio				
Yes	212	98,6	149	100,0
No	3	1,4	0	0,0
Tuberculosis				
Yes	93	43,3	93	62,4
No	122	56,7	56	37,6
Diphtheria				
Yes	4	1,9	10	6,7
No	211	98,1	139	93,3
Tetanus				
Yes	102	47,4	80	53,7
No	113	52,6	69	46,3
Whooping cough				
Yes	19	8,8	16	10,7
No	196	91,2	133	89,3
Hepatitis B				
Yes	7	3,3	5	3,4
No	208	96,7	144	96,6
Pneumonia				
Yes	13	6,0	9	6,0
No	202	94,0	140	94,0
Meningitis				
Yes	11	5,1	11	7,4
No	201	93,5	138	92,6
Measles				
Yes	198	92,1	147	98,7
No	17	7,9	2	1,3
Yellow Fever				
Yes	120	55,8	117	78,5
No	95	44,2	32	21,5

Table XII shows that the proportion of mothers of children aged 12 to 23 months who did not recognise certain VRE (poliomyelitis, tuberculosis, diphtheria, tetanus, whooping cough, meningitis, measles and yellow fever) was higher in the ENCV than in the ENCV. It shows that a mother's lack of awareness of VEMs is associated with failure to complete the child's immunisation schedule.

Table XIII. Knowledge of mothers responsible for children aged 12 to 23 months about the different vaccines used in routine EPI

	Fully vaccinated children			
Vaccines	No		Yes	
	210	%	152	%
BCG				
Yes	115	54,8	128	84,2
No	95	45,2	24	15,8
VPO				
Yes	187	89,0	147	96,7
No	23	11,0	5	3,3
DTP-HepB-Hib				
Yes	22	10,5	18	11,8
No	188	89,5	134	88,2
PCV-13				
Yes	0	0,0	6	3,9
No	210	100,0	146	96,1
VAA				
Yes	103	49,0	127	83,6
No	107	51,0	25	16,4
VAR				
Yes	179	85,2	141	92,8
No	31	14,8	11	7,2

Table XIII shows that the proportion of mothers of children aged 12 to 23 months who had no knowledge of the vaccines used at the SPC was higher in the ENCVs than in the ECVs.

Table XIV. Main sources of information on vaccination for mothers responsible for children aged 12 to 23 months.

Fully vaccinated children				
sources of information	No		Yes	
	n= 215	%	n = 152	%
Medical staff	37	17,2	58	38,2
Community relay	30	14,0	41	27,0
Church	14	6,5	2	1,3
Radio	6	2,8	6	3,9
Television	40	18,6	15	9,9
Town crier	88	40,9	28	18,4
Other sources	2	0,9	2	1,3

Table XIV shows that the main channels of communication for ENCV mothers were: Cries (40.9 Vs 18.4), Television (18.6 Vs 9.9) and Church (6.5 Vs 1.3), while for ECV mothers the main channels were: medical staff (38.2 Vs 17.2), Community Relais (27.0 Vs 14.0) and Radio (3.9 Vs 2.8).

Table XV: The main reasons for not vaccinating, in descending order, mothers who have not completed the immunisation schedule for their children aged 12 to 23 months in the Bandalungwa health zone, 2016.

N°	Reasons for not vaccinating	N	Workforce	Proportion
1	Social occupations	367	160	43,8%
2	Lack information	367	100	27,4%
3	Vaccine unavailability	367	93	25,5%
4	Fear of side effects	367	52	14,2%
5	Didn't know where to go	367	15	4,1%
6	Religious beliefs	367	14	3,8%
7	Long waiting times	367	12	3,3%
8	Lack confidence in staff	367	8	2,2%
9	Remote structures	367	5	1,4%

Table XV shows that social occupations followed by lack of information (43.8%, 27.4%) are the main reasons why children are not vaccinated.

3.5. Determinants of non-completion of the vaccination schedule

The determinants of non-completion of the vaccination schedule derived from the bivariate analysis of each independent variable with the dependent variable (non-completion of the vaccination schedule in children aged 12 to 23 months) and from the multivariate analysis in the logistic regression model.

1. Determinants of non-completion of the vaccination schedule in bivariate analysis

Table XVI: Socio-demographic characteristics of mothers associated with non-completion of the immunisation schedule for children aged 12 to 23 months, Bandalungwa Health Zone, 2016

Fully vaccinated children							
					OR	95% CI	p
Determinants	No		Yes				
	n= 215	%	n= 152	%			
Age of mothers							
≤24 (young people)	52	24,2	26	17,1	0,64	[3,8 ; 1,09]	0,102
≥25Adulites	163	75,8	126	82,9			
Level of education							
High level	22	10,2	25	16,4	0,58	[0,313 ; 1,071	0,79
Low level	193	89,8	127	83,6			
Profession							
Housekeeper	67	31,1	52	34,2	0,87	[0,56 ; 1,35]	0,094
Non-household	148	68,9	100	65,8			
Marital status							
In union	54	25,1	27	17,8	0,64	[0,38; 1,08]	0,094
Single	161	74,9	125	82,2			
child's sex							
Male	105	48,3	96	63,2	1,8	[1,18 ; 2,75]	0,007*
Female	110	51,7	56	36,8			

Table XIV of the bivariate analysis shows that only the female sex of the child is statistically significantly associated with non-completion of the vaccination schedule for children aged 12 to 23 months, p= 0.007. Among children not fully vaccinated, the female sex is significantly predominant (66.3%) over the male sex (52.2%).

Table XVII: Knowledge, attitude, organisation of vaccination service, geographical and financial accessibility.

Fully vaccinated children							
	No		Yes		OR	95% CI	p
Determinants	Number of employees, n= 215	%	Number of employees, n= 152	%			
Level of knowledge							
Acceptable	134	62,3	106	69,7	1,4	[0,89; 2,10]	0,142
low	81	37,7	46	30,3			
Attitude of mothers face to the vaccination							
Good	31	20,4	98	45,6	1,4	[0,51 ; 3,74]	0,515
Wrong	121	79,6	117	54,4	1		
Possession of the card							
Yes	62	28,8	150	98,7	185	[44,47 ; 770]	0,00*
No	153	71,2	2	1,3	1		
Waiting time to service of vaccination							
≤ 1 hour	73	34,0	82	53,9	2,3	[1,47 ; 3,46]	0,00*
> 1 hour	141	66,0	70	46,1	1		
History of MAPI							
No	90	41,9	75	49,3	1,4	[0,89 ; 2,05]	0,163
Yes	125	58,1	77	50,7	1		
Welcome to the vaccination site							
Good	168	78,1	152	100,0	1,9	[1,21 2,11]	0,00*
Bad	47	21,9	0	0,0	1		
Assessment of the cost of the session of the CPS							
Normal	101	47,0	124	81,6	2,0	[1,12 3,32]	0,00*
High	114	53,0	28	18,4	1		
Distance from vaccination site							
≤ 30 minutes walking distance	132	61,4	140	92,1	7,33	[3, 82;14,0]	0,00*
> 30 minutes walking distance	83	38,6	12	7,9			
API index							
High	137	63,7	105	69,0	0,78	[0,50 ; 1,22]	0,286
Low	78	36,3	47	31,0			

Bivariate analysis of table XVII shows that the non-availability of the vaccination card, long waiting times at CPS sessions, poor reception at the vaccination service, the high cost of the vaccination service and the long distance to the vaccination site were statistically associated with non-completion of the vaccination schedule for children aged 12 to 23 months in the Bandalungwa health zone.

The proportion of mothers who did not make the card available was higher for ENCVs than for ECVs (71.2 Vs 1.3). Non-completion of the vaccination calendar was one hundred and eighty times more associated with the availability of the vaccination card among respondents (p= 0.00).

The proportion of mothers who felt that the waiting time at the CPS was longer in the ENCVs compared to the ECVs (66.0 Vs 41.1).Non-completion of the vaccination schedule was two point three more associated with waiting time at the CPS session. (p=0,00).

Non-completion of the vaccination schedule was twice associated with the high cost of HPC (p=0.00). The proportion of mothers who felt that the cost of HPC was higher in ENCVs than in ECVs (53.3 vs 18.4).

Finally, non-completion of the vaccination schedule was seven times more associated with mothers who walked more than 30 minutes from home to the vaccination site (p=0.00). The proportion of mothers who felt that they walked more than 30 minutes from home to the vaccination site in the NCVS group was greater than in the ECV group (38.6 Vs 7.9).

Table XVIII: Determinants of non-completion of the vaccination schedule for children aged 12 to 23 months.

Determinants	OR Gross	95% CI	p	OR adjusted	95% CI	p
Possession of the card						
Yes	1					
No	185	[44,47 ; 770,00]	< 0,0001 *	144,1	[33,74 ; 615,74]	0,000*
Waiting times at the CPS						
< 1 hour	1					
≥ 1 hour	2,26	[1,47 ; 3,46]	< 0,0001 *	2,19	[1,17 ; 4,11]	0,014*
Welcome to CS						
Good	1					
Bad	1,9	[1,21 ; 2,11]	< 0,0001 *	0,98	[0,56 ; 2, 29]	0,56
Cost of the CPS session						
Normal	1					
High	7,33	[3,82 ; 14,0]	< 0,0001 *	4,21	[2,33 ; 6,75]	0,006*
Child's gender						
Male	1					
Female	1,8	[1,18; 2,75]	0,007*			

After introducing the six variables associated with non-completion of the immunisation schedule in bivariate analysis, logistic regression was used to identify the following as determinants of non-completion of the immunisation schedule in children aged 12 to 23 months: non-availability of the immunisation card, long waiting times for mothers at the CPS session, and the high cost of the CPS session.

CHAPTER IV

DISCUSSION

This study enabled us to identify the determinants of non-completion of the vaccination schedule, namely: the availability of the vaccination card, the long waiting at the vaccination session and the high cost of the CPS session.

4.1. VACCINATION COVERAGE

The proportion of fully vaccinated children found overall was 41.4± 7% (IC95% 34.4-48.4), well below that reported in the provincial city of Kinshasa according to the DHS 2013-2014 report (68%, IC95%: 62-74) (4) but close to that of the DRC. This difference can be explained by the fluctuation in the sample size, went 35 ZS in the provincial city of Kinshasa to the ZS of Bandalungwa.In addition, we collected information from mothers responsible for children aged 12 to 23 months in two ways: according to the vaccination card, which is perfectly certain, and according to mothers' declarations, whose reliability may be questioned. In our study, 57.8 ± 7% (IC95% 50.8-64.8) of mothers had the vaccination card, whereas in the 2013-2014 DHS report for the city of Kinshasa, only 44% of children had made the vaccination card available (4).

4.2. Mothers' knowledge and attitudes to vaccination

In our study, we found that the proportion of mothers with a low level of knowledge (unable to cite: 5MEVs, one benefit of vaccination, one consequence of vaccination and 5 appointments in the vaccination calendar) was higher among ENCVs than ECVs (37.7 Vs 30.3) and 57.8 ± 7% (IC95% 50.8-64.8) had made the vaccination card available. And 65% of mothers had a good attitude to vaccination. The low level of knowledge has been found in several studies of non-completion of the childhood vaccination schedule (34, 35, 36, 37, 39). Our results on mothers' knowledge of vaccination are similar to those reported by Kiyimbi **(33)**.This can be explained by the fact that mothers in the DRC all have almost the same level of information about vaccination, as source of communication is the same and the level of literacy is almost equal throughout the DRC's female community.This low level of knowledge among mothers about vaccination could be explained by the deterioration in the quality of education in the country and the declining level of literacy among young women. Regarding mothers' attitudes to vaccination, we found that 79.6% of ENCV mothers had poor vaccination habits, compared with 54.4% of ECV mothers. These results corroborate those found by certain authors. (33,43)

4.3. Determinants of non-completion of the vaccination schedule for children aged 12 to 23 months.

After bi-variate analyses, we found that six factors were significantly associated with non-completion of the vaccination schedule for children aged 12 to 23 months, namely: non-availability of the vaccination card, long waiting time at the vaccination site, poor reception at the vaccination site, high cost of the vaccination session, distance of more than 30 minutes' walk to the vaccination site and female gender.After logistic regression analysis of these six variables, only three were retained as determinants of non-completion of the vaccination schedule for children aged 12 to 23 months in the Bandalungwa health zone:

1. Availability of the vaccination card

Using bivariate analysis and logistic regression, we found that non-availability of the card was associated with non-completion of the immunisation schedule for children aged 12 to 23 (0R = 144.1, IC95% [33.74; 615.74]; p =0.00). Several studies have found similar results: Ndeye M et al in Senegal, Odusanya O et col. in Nigeria, and Kiyimbi and Kahozi in the DRC (23, 26, 33, 43).

2. Waiting time at the vaccination site

According to our results, waiting times of more than one hour were associated with children not completing their vaccination schedule (OR = 2.19, IC95% [1.17; 4.11]); p= 0.014). This situation could be improved in the routine EPI reinforcement approach by increasing the supervision of the structures that vaccinate. Some authors have also suggested this in their studies, such as Baonga and Kiyimbi (33, 34).

3. Cost of the CPS session

Most of the mothers who did not complete the vaccination schedule for their children aged 12 to 23 months were faced with the high cost of the vaccination session given their low financial income (0R = 4.21, IC95% [2.33; 6.75], p = 0.006). These results are similar to those reported by LINK-GELLES R and al (29).

4.4. Strengths and limitations of study

a) Force

Our study had the privilege of highlighting the proportion of ECVs according to information obtained from mothers responsible for children aged 12 to 23 in the Bandalungwa health zone. These results could, on the one hand, guide decision-makers in terms of vaccination and, on the other hand, help the structures in charge to ensure that children are vaccinated, so that they understand that the health of the population is their responsibility, and to involve the community in all the strategies envisaged to improve vaccination coverage in the Bandalungwa HZ.

b) Limits

Our study has a number of limitations:

• The study population is a sample drawn from the general population, although there may be some irregularities in the representativeness of the population, as low vaccination coverage is reported in 12 of the 35 Kinshasa health zones, whereas we have restricted our study to just one health zone.

• The information obtained from the declarations of mothers who did not have vaccination cards for their children was taken with reservations, as the reliability of the information is questionable and may introduce information bias (memory bias).

• The very limited number of variables that were statistically significant does not necessarily guarantee vaccination coverage in the health zone. However, our study remains open to further investigation by others, based on the limited information we were able to obtain.

CONCLUSION AND RECOMMENDATIONS

To conclude our study, we note that the proportion of ECVs in the Bandalungwa health zone remains low. The main reasons why children aged between 12 and 23 months do not complete their vaccination schedule are: the unavailability of the vaccination card, the long waiting time for mothers at the vaccination site and the high cost of the CPS session.

In view of the above, we recommend :

1. At the EPI (Management, Kinshasa Coordination and the Kinshasa West branch)

• To make the vaccination cards available in the health zone so that each mother can obtain them during the vaccination session in order to guarantee real information on EPI activities.
• Increase the number of channels for communicating about immunisation, so that the population takes ownership of it and puts their children's immunisation activities at the forefront, enabling the programme to achieve its objectives.

2. To the Bandalungwa ZS and all its staff

• To improve the quality of the vaccination service at all levels, so that the long waiting time and high cost of the vaccination session do not constitute a barrier for mothers to have their children vaccinated.

3. To the mothers responsible for children aged 12 to 23 months and to the entire Bandalungwa ZS community

• Keep their children's vaccination cards so that they don't lose information about vaccinations and even about keeping appointments;
• To understand that their children's health is a priority above all else, because the long waiting time and the fees they are asked to pay at the CPS meeting are not a barrier to completing their children's vaccination schedule.
• To become more involved in promoting the health of their children in particular and of everyone in general.

BIBLIOGRAPHICAL REFERENCES

1. WHO, Vaccine-preventable diseases bulletin, Geneva, Fact sheet September 2016;

2. WHO, Immunization coverage, Fact sheet No. 378, Multimedia Centre, Geneva, September 2015 ;

3. WHO, Vaccination coverage, Fact sheet, Geneva, September 2016

4. Rapport 2013-2014, RDC, Enquête Démographique et de Santé, Ministère du Plan et Suivi de la Mise en œuvre de la Révolution de la Modernité and Ministère de la Santé Publique, République Démocratique du Congo, 2014 edition.

5. Mapatano et al,Immunisation-related knowledge, attitudes and practices of mothers in Kinshasa, Democratic Republic of the Congo.SA Fam Pract,2008

6. Programme Elargie de Vaccination, Democratic Republic of Congo, annual report 2015, PEV/RCD, unpublished, February 2016

7. WHO, Democratic Republic of Congo, Rapport d'analyse des résultats des activités du PEV de routine dans la ville province de Kinshasa au premier semestre 2014, unpublished, 2015

8. NIAID-National Institute of Allergy and Infection Diseases-dossier Acrobat Reader produced by NIAID "Understanding Vaccines :What they are - How they work"- US Department of Health and human services - NIH publication N0.03-4219-July 2003

9. Expanded Programme on Immunisation: 25 years tomorrow. Med. Trop, 2001,61, 177-186

10. WHO, Unicef: Vaccines and immunization, the world situation, Geneva 1996).

11. Lambert PH ; Liu M ; Siegrist CA ; Revue Pratique : Immunité anti-infectieuse : mécanismes, facteurs spécifiques et non spécifiques. 1994; 44: 2505- (WHORoutine immunization coverage worldwide).

12. Jacqueline Etienne ; Eric Clauser : Biochimie Génétique - Biologie Moléculaire - 7ème édition - Masson, Paris, 1987, 2001 - Masson S.A - 120, Boulevard Saint Germain - 75 280 Paris Cedex 06 - (p370-371)

13. Brien Fitzgibbon ; 1,2 Laurie Ackermann ; 1,4 Kevin Murphy ; Michel Deming ; 1 Jacqueline Gindler3 : Expanded Programme on Immunisation (EPI) in 12 African countries 1982 - 1993.

14. Rapport Programme élargie de vaccination (PEV), plan pluri annuelle 2015-2019, unpublished, PEV.RDC, 2015.

15. Vulgaris médical: medical knowledge in a language accessible to all

16. HUG Pharmacy website - http://pharmacie.hug-ge.ch/ Information on medicines - Recommendations for use Pharmaceutical assistance: internal tel. 31080).

17. Bos, E., and Batson, A. Using immunization coverage rates for monitoring health sector performance: Measurement and interpretation issues. Washington DC: Human development network, The World Bank; 2000, 1-21.)

18. Fairbrother, G., Freed, G. L., and Thompson, J. W. Measuring immunization coverage.Amer J Prev Med. 2000;19(3 Suppl):78-88.

19. Bolton, P., Hussain, A., Hadpawat, A., Holt, E., Hughart, N., etGuyer, B. Deficiencies in current childhood immunization indicators. Public Health Rep. 1998; 113(6):527- 32.)

20. Expanded Programme on Immunization (EPI) in 12 African countries 1982 - 1993Brian Fitzgibbon, 1,2 Laurie Ackerman, I, 4 Kevin Murphy Michael Deming,1 Jacqueline Gindler3.)

21. Gianluca Russo1 and all; Vaccine coverage and determinants of incomplete vaccination in children aged 12-23 months in Dschang, West Region, Cameroon: a cross-sectional survey during a polio outbreak vol 33, n°7, 2009, p.43-49.

22. Faye A., Seck I., Dia A.T., Facteurs d'abandon de la vaccination en milieu Rural Sénégal, Médecine d'Afrique noire, vol 57,n°3,2010, p.137-141.

23. Ndeye M.N., Ndiaye P., Abdoulaye D., et al, Facteurs d'abandon de la vaccination des enfants âgés de 10 à 23 mois à Ndoulo (Sénégal), Cahier d'étude et de recherche francophone/Santé, Volume 19, Numéro 1,2009.

24. Aicha Hamid; Evaluation de la couverture vaccinale des jeunes enfants de la Montérégie au regard des facteurs sociodémographiques et impact de l'ajout de nouveaux vaccins, June 2008, vol 21, page 20-25.

25. BeckieNnenna Tagbo1,2, et al, Vaccination Coverage and Its Determinants in Children Aged 11 - 23 Months in an Urban District of Nigeria; vol 49, p 19-23

26. Olumuyiwa O Odusanya, Ewan F Alufohai, Francois P Maurice and Vincent I, determinants of vaccination coverage in rural Nigeria. BMC Public Health 2008Ahonkhai. 8:381 doi: 10.1186/1471-2458-8- 381;

27. Rapport Programme Elargie de vaccination (PEV) Benin, Revue externe 2008, Rapport Inédit, Cotonou, Mars 2009 ;

28. Dr. Kaïdtlila nenouara and Prof. Glangeaud Jean Paul, la situation vaccinale des enfants en période du P.A.S. en Algérie, résultats d'une enquête auprès des ménages de la wilaya de Bejaia ; vol 79, p 98-106.

29. Link-Gelles R et al. A national survey of obstetricians about attitudes on maternal and

infant immunization. Emergnence response research center, Atlanta, 2011.vol 12,p 14-17

30. Rapport de Programme Elargie de vaccination (PEV) Côte d'Ivoire ; Revue externe, Abidjan, Rapport Inédit. 2008.

31. Final Report. Maputo, Ministry of Health, Expanded Program on Immunization, Mozambique: A Study to Describe Barriers to Childhood Vaccination in Mozambique. F; the CHANGE Project, and Project HOPE, Sheldon SJ, C Alons. July 2003.

32. Report on the Expanded Programme on Immunisation (EPI): External Review. Unpublished report. Ndjamena, April 2012 ;

33. Kiyimbi Bushidi Pontien. Déterminants de non achèvement du calendrier vaccinal des enfants de 12 à 23 mois dans la ZS de Muanda, Dissertation, ESP/Kinshasa 2012.

34. Baonga BA POUTH Simon Franky et al.Vaccine coverage and factors associated with vaccine non-completeness in children aged 12 to 23 months in the Djoungolo-Cameroon health district in 2012, Published: 04/11/2016.Available on internet: http://www.panafrican-med-journal.com/content/article/17/91/full

35. Verger Pierre, Attitude et pratiques des médecins généralistes de la ville relatives à la vaccination en général et celle de la grippe en 2009.Panel, 2011.

36. Ouedraogo L.T et al. Determinants of non-compliance with the immunisation schedule of the Expanded Programme on Immunisation at health district level: the case of the health district of Boussé, Burkina-Faso .Médecine et maladies infectieuses, 2006.

37. Nankabirwa V, TYLLESKAR T, TUMWINE JK et al. Maternal education is associated with vaccination status of infants less than 6 months in Eastern Uganda: a cohort study. PubMed 2010.

38. Mollema L, Wijers N, Haline, Vander Klis. Participation and attitude towards the national immunization program in Netherlands. BMC Public Health, 2012.

39. Batumbo Boloweti. Evaluation sur le niveau de connaissance, les attitudes ainsi que les pratiques des mères d'enfants de 0 à 23 mois dans la ZS de santé de Ngabavis-à-vis de la vaccination, Dissertation, ESP/Kinshasa,2013.

40. Rimple D, Weiss SJ, Brett M, Ernest A. An emergency department based vaccination program: Overcocoming the barriers for adults at high risk for vaccine preventable diseases. Acad Emerg Med. September 2006

41. Matango CLUB. The situation of children in the world: the case of Cameroon, 2014, available on the Internet: http://matango.mondoblog.org/2014/06/18/la-situation- des-enfants-dans-le-monde-le-cas-du-cameroun

42. Rapport Annuel Direction d'Etude et Planification (DEP-RDC), Ministry of Public

Health, Unpublished report, 2012.

43. Kaozi Mihali, facteurs associés la non complétude du calendrier vaccinal des enfants de 12 à 23 mois dans la ZS de BARUMBU, Dissertation, ESP/Kinshasa 2014.

APPENDICES

APPENDIX I: INFORMATION FOR INFORMED CONSENT

Mr, Mrs

I am MUSA WABULA Moise, a student at the School of Public Health at the University of Kinshasa in the 2nd year of a Master's degree in Intervention Epidemiology and Laboratory Management. I am conducting this study on "the determinants of non-completion of the immunisation schedule in children aged 13 to 23 and in mothers carrying children aged 0 to 11 months in the Bandalungwa Health Zone, City of Kinshasa. This study was carried out in the DRC for my dissertation. The aim of this study is to determine the factors associated with low vaccination coverage in the Bandalungwa health zone from 1 January 2015 to 30 June 2016.This health zone has had low coverage of all antigens (see 2014 and 2015 EPI annual reports) and reported a number of cases of vaccine-preventable diseases in 2014-2015 (according to a WHO survey on vaccination coverage), with a high risk of epidemic outbreaks in the coming days.We will guarantee the strictly scientific nature of study and the data obtained will be kept strictly confidential.To signify your consent to this study, please sign the form attached to this information note.Thank you for your time.

APPENDIX II: DATA COLLECTION TOOLS

Vaccination coverage children aged 12 to 23 months

	Province: Kinshasa			Bandalungwa health zone				Areao f health/ quartier :							
	Bunch No: ///		Date of ////	the survey	:	Time	from	start:							
N° of the menage	N° of the child	Vaccination card (+,-)	Date Child's date of birth (Day/month/year)		Vaccinations received: enter the date (day/month/year) and place (Pu=public centre, Pr=private centre, Cf=denominational centre) of all vaccinations.										
				BC G (date/place)	Cicatrice BCG (+,-,A)	Polio zero(date/place)	Polio 1 (date/place)	Polio 2 (date/place)	Polio 3 (date/place)	Pentavalent 1 (date/lieu)	Pentavalent 2 (date/lieu)	Pentavalent 3 (date/lieu)	PCV-13	VAR (date/place)	VAA (date/place)

SURVEY ON THE KNOWLEDGE, ATTITUDES AND PRACTICES IN THE DEBANDALUNGWA HEALTH ZONE

QUESTIONNAIRE

Household identification: Id COLLECTION INFORMATION: RC

RC1. Name of investigator:|RC2. Supervisor's NAMEI|

RC3. Day/Month/Year of interview:2_|_0_|_1_|_6_|

After completing household interview, fill in the following information:

RC5. Result of interview:.RC6A. Responsibility of the respondent in the household

1=Completely filled 2=Partially filled 3=Refused

4=Other to be specified

RC6B. GENDER OF RESPONDENT IN HOUSEHOLD (M/F):

RC8. Number children aged 12-23 months:

1. HOUSEHOLD CHARACTERISTICS: CM

N°	Questions	Answers and Codes	
CM1	In what months and years were you born? completed)	/..../.../.../.../..../...../ NSP 98 No answer 99	| |
CM02	What is the respondent's marital status?	Marie in monogamy1 Marie in polygamy2 Single 3 Divorcee/Separate/widow4 Common-law union5 Other to be specified6	| |
CM03	Which is Your level of education (Have you been school?)	Primary1 Secondary 2 Higher/University 3 None 4	| |
CM04	What do you do for a living?	Menagere1 Retailer2 Civil servant3 Civil servant4 No profession5 Other to be specified6	| |
CM05	What is your current religion?	No religion1 Catholic2 Protestant3 Kimbanguist4 Muslim woman 5 Eglise de reveil 6 Jehovah's Witness7 Other to be specified8	| |
CM06	What is your relationship with the Head of Household?	Head of housekeeping 1 Spouse of head of household2 Child of the house3 PARENTS OF A SPOUSE 4 SISTER, COUSINE, NIECE FROM ONE FROM SPOUSE 5 Others to be specified 6	| |
CM07	How many of	/..../..../	
	people live at your home		
CM08	How much do you spend average per day on eat (convert to Dollars)	/........../	

<table>
<tr><td rowspan="2">CM09</td><td rowspan="2">Do you own?</td><td rowspan="2">Tap water In the household Internal toilet Electricity PERMANENT Vehicle Television flat screen Refrigerator AISON EN CARREAUX</td><td>YES</td><td>NO</td><td></td></tr>
<tr><td>1
1
1
1
1
1
1
1</td><td>0
0
0
0
0
0
0
0</td><td></td></tr>
<tr><td>CM10</td><td>The birth of your children aged 12-23 months were done where?</td><td colspan="3">Home 1
Training health 2
Home and training 3
SANITARY</td><td>| |</td></tr>
</table>

2. IDENTIFICATION OF CHILDREN AND THEIR VACCINATIONS

IDENTIFICATION AND VACCINATION OF CHILDREN: IEV			
IEV01	Child's gender	Male...1 Feminine...2			
ENI02	Child's age (in completed months)	Date of birth ..../........../			
IEV03	Has the child been fully vaccinated?	Yes1 No.2			
IEV04	If the child has not had all the vaccinations, what are the reasons? (Three choices)	Lack of information and communication 11 Fear of side effects 12 Religious beliefs13 Fear of witchcraft14 Didn't know where to get vaccinated15 Distance from health facilities21 Economic activities22 Social obligations/household23 Not a decision-maker within the family24 Lack of trust in healthcare staff. 31 Lack of financial resources32 Unavailability of vaccines...33 Waiting time too long, bad welcome.34 Other (please specify)... 55		||
IEV05	At what age should your child be vaccinated against measles and yellow fever?	Don't know1 9thmonth2 Other (please specify)3			
IEV06	Who in the household makes the decision about vaccination?	Father1 Mother 2 Grandparents3 Other (please specify)5			
IEV07	When do you usually have your child vaccinated? (First three answers)	At birth 1 Depending on the Appointment2 When he's ill and I take him to hospital 3 During campaigns4 When there is an epidemic5 Other (please specify)6		
IEV08	What prompted you to have your children vaccinated at these particular times?	Keeping to schedule/RDV1 Opportunit2 Social mobilisation3 Other 4			

3. MOTHERS' KNOWLEDGE OF VACCINATION

N°	Questions	Answers			Codes
CMV 1	Is there a service vaccination at your country?	No...1 Yes2 DK3			| |
CMV 2	Has your child been vaccinated?	No...1 Yes2			| |
CMV 3	If yes, where did you follow the vaccination	In the commune...1 outside the commune...2			| |
CMV 4	Have you ever heard of vaccine	No...1 Yes2			| |
CMV 5	What is your main source of information on vaccination?	medical staff1 the community relay2 the church3 the radio...4 Television5 town crier6 other to be specified7			| |
CMV 6	How important do you think it is to have your child vaccinated?	Protection1 Growing up well2 DK3			| |
CMV 7	Do you know the consequences if your child is not vaccinated?	The disease1 Disability... 2 Dying3 Others to be specified4 DK5			| |
			YES	NO	
CMV 8	Do you know which diseases children are vaccinated against? (several answers possible)	Poliomyelitis Tuberculosis Diphtheria Tetanus Whooping cough Hepatitis Pneumonia Meningitis	1 1 1 1 1 1 1 1	0 0 0 0 0 0 0 0	
		Measles Yellow fever Don't know	1 1 1	0 0 0	
CMV 9	What do you do when your child catches these diseases?	Nothing...0 I care at home1 I'm taking him to hospital2 I go church3 I go traditional			| |

		practitioners...4 Others to be specified 5			
CMV 10	How many times have you take your child to the health centre for vaccination	None0 once1 more than ...2			| |
CMV 11	List the vaccinations your child should have		YES	NO	
		BCG	1	0	
		VPO	1	0	
		DTC-	1	0	
		HepB-	1	0	
		Hib	1	0	
		PCV-13	1	0	
		VAA	1	0	
		VAR DK	1	0	
CMV 12	At what age should a child be vaccinated?	At birth...1 At 1 and a half months2 At 2 and a half months3 At 3 and a half months4 At 9 months5 DK6			| |

4. MOTHERS' ATTITUDES TO VACCINATION

AMV 1	How dodo you consider the vaccine	Dangerous 1 Non-hazardous 2 DK 3	
AMV 2	Do you think the vaccine can protect your child	No...0 Yes1 DK98	| || |
AMV 3	If your vaccination site is about a 45-minute away, can you to go	No...0 Yes1	| |
AMV 4	How do you feel if your child is vaccinated?	1=Satisfied1 2=concerned...2 3=Nothing3 4=Other to be specified4 98= DK98	| |
AMV 5	What motivates you to go and vaccinate your child?	prevent it falling ill 1 By this that the other the do the community relay...2 Hospital demands3 Radio...4 Television...5 Others to be specified6 DK98	| |
AMV 6	How do you assess the seriousness of vaccine-preventable diseases?	Grave/Mortelles1 Less serious2 Others to be specified3 DK98	| |
AMV 7	Are you satisfied with the results of the vaccination	No...1 Yes2 DK98	| |
AMV 8	If not, why not	the child the fever1 the child falls ill2 Others to be specified3	| |

5. ORGANISING VACCINATION SERVICES

N°	Questions	Answers and Codes			
OSV 1	On average, how long do you wait at the CS for your child to is vaccinated	/......./...../minutes			
OSV 2	At any time in the past, has your child had any symptoms after receiving vaccinations?	No... 1 Yes 2 DK 98			| |
OSV 3	If so, which ones?	Fever Abscess Shock Acute flaccid paralysis Convulsion Death Others to be specified........	YES	NO	
			1 1 1 1 1 1 1 1 1	0 0 0 0 0 0 0 0 0	
OSV 4	How do you rate the welcome at CS	Bad 1 So... 2			| |
OSV 5	Has your child ever missed a vaccination due to a shortage of CS vaccine?	Yes 1 No... 2 DK98			| |
OSV 6	Has your child ever missed a vaccination due to the repeated absence of CS staff?	Yes1 No...2 DK3			| |

6. GEOGRAPHICAL AND FINANCIAL ACCESSIBILITY

N°	Questions	Answers and Codes	
AGFV 1	How much walking do you do to the vaccination site	Less than hour...1 Over an hour... 2			
AGFV 2	The sessions of vaccination paid for?	Yes 1 No... 2 DK98			
AGFV 3	Yes, what is the price per session	Minus $1.1 More than $1.2			
AGFV 4	How do you assess the cost of vaccination	High... 1 Normal 2			

Thank you for your kind contribution

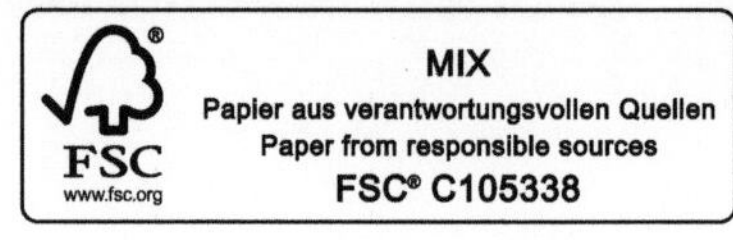

Printed by Books on Demand GmbH, Norderstedt / Germany